HOW TO STAY SANE

IN AN

INSANE COVID-WORLD

HOW TO STAY SANE

IN AN

INSANE COVID-WORLD

How to cope with the stress of a COVID pandemic, a (partial) lockdown, working from home and videoconferencing.

Dr Theo Compernolle MD., PhD.

COMPUBLICATIONS
SCIENCE MADE SIMPEL AND USEFUL

About the author

<u>Dr Theo Compernolle</u> MD. PhD Is a neuropsychiatrist who teaches and coaches in the executive programs of business schools including CEDEP in France. IMD in Switzerland and TIAS in the Netherlands.
He also consults, teaches and coaches professionals, managers and executives in a wide range of (multi)national companies, professional services firms and training institutions in many different cultures and countries.
He holds these sessions in English, Dutch and French.

Before, he has held the positions of Suez Chair in Leadership and Personal Development at the Solvay Business School, Adjunct Professor at INSEAD, visiting professor at several business schools and Professor at the Free University of Amsterdam.

As a medical doctor, neuropsychiatrist, psychotherapist and business consultant, Theo studies research from very different fields including medicine, biology, psychology, neurology, physiology and management.
He then burns the midnight oil to integrate this information into a coherent whole and to find simple ways to pass on this knowledge, in a memorable way, to all kinds of professionals.
He has published several non-fiction books and more than a hundred scientific articles. Three of his books ao. *"STRESS: FRIEND AND FOE"* and *"BRAINCHAINS"* became bestsellers

More information at www.comperrnolle.com
Contact: form@compernoplle.org

Table of contents

Introduction

Since we got in the depth of this Corona pandemic I received a lot of questions from clients, people as well as companies, about how to deal with this unusual stress-situation. Although the situation is unique, we can learn from a lot of research from many different fields about how to cope with it.

In a pandemic there are lots of terrible and tragic events that are outside of your control. To stay sane in such an insane world it is important to choose your battles wisely and to concentrate on the many things you can do within your niche of control.

Moreover, Since working from home is here to stay for many of us, we might as well learn from what the lockdown home-work pressure cooker forced upon us.

Let me summarize the core issues and give you a few solutions.

Good luck!
In French people say "Bon courage!" which means "Good courage". You probably will need both.
Theo Compernolle

PS. I wrote an article about "Long Covid" or "Post Acute Sequelae of COVID" for family physicians.
You can find a quick and dirty English translation at www.compernolle.com tab: Free texts.
There you will also find a summary of my books *"Stress: Friend and Foe"* and *"BrainChains"* and other texts that may be interesting for you.

1. <u>How To Keep Your Stress-Balance</u>

Stress can harm people and organizations, but stress also helps us to be creative and deliver top performance. The

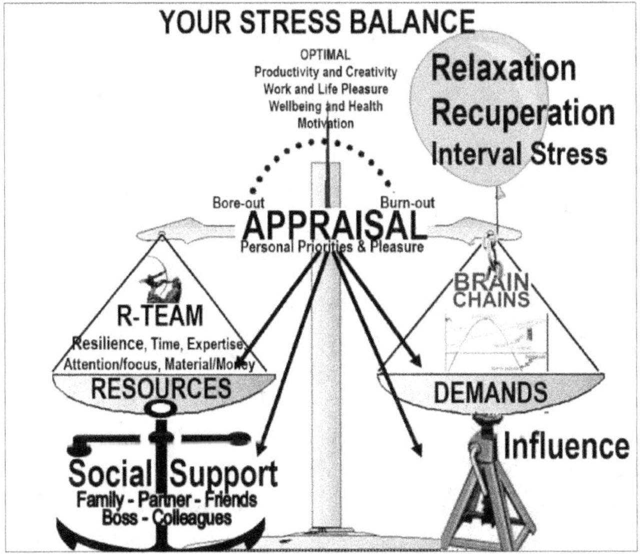

best metaphor for what stress actually is, is a bow. The stress in the bow gives the arrow the energy needed to reach the goal! Without stress in the bow, the arrow gets nowhere. However, if the bow is over-tensioned, it loses its resilience. The same happens if one forgets to "de-span" the bow after use! So there is positive and negative, healthy and unhealthy stress, stimulating and paralyzing stress, fantastic stress and deadly stress, eu-stress and dis-stress.

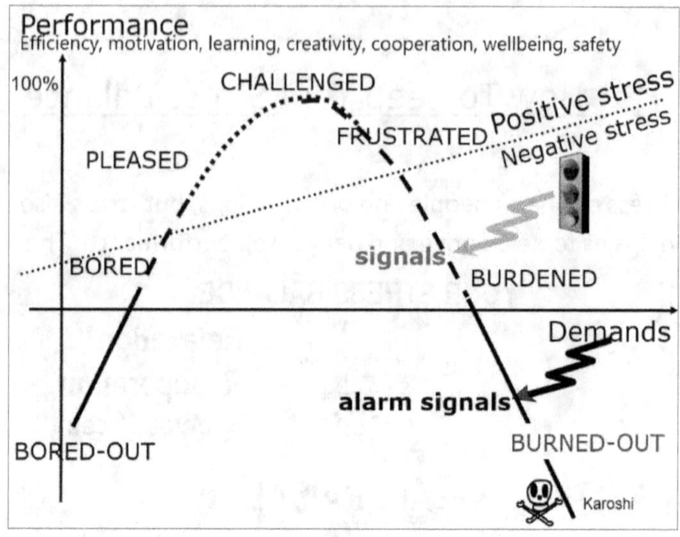

So the question is not: how do I prevent stress, but how do I keep my stress as a friend.

To summarize the hundreds of thousands of research publications on stress, I always use the image of the stress scale and balance. The stress scale and balance remind you that there are six core factors that you should always consider as a possible cause of imbalance. They are also the key to restoring the imbalance: the demands, the resources, social support, influence, time for recovery, and our interpretation of those five elements.

The concept of scale and balance shows that even if the factor that caused the imbalance cannot be influenced, such as an epidemic, the imbalance can still be restored through action in other areas. "Being in balance" also makes it clear that the level of demands is not a problem in itself, as long as it is in balance with the other five factors.

In general, you can try to restore your stress balance by starting to ask yourself a few questions (these are extensively discussed in my book "Stress: Friend and Foe". The English version exhausted. A fourth and total revision will be available in Q1 of 2022, but you can also find a summary on www.compernolle.com tab: free text.

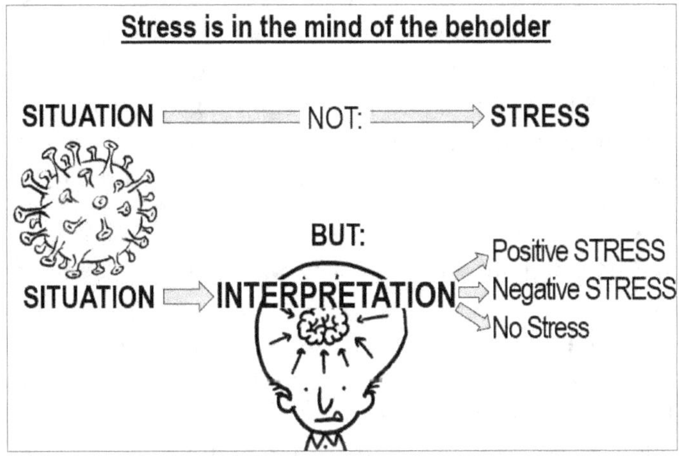

Stress Is In The Eye Of The Beholder

A key question is: **how do you look at the situation**? It is often the most important question because your interpretation of the situation largely determines what and how you feel and what you do or do not do. Your interpretation of the situation is key and central to your stress balance. The same stress situation can be judged and interpreted differently by different people as irrelevant, as a threat, as a challenge, as an aggression, or as a pleasure. They will react differently to it: with indifference, with fear, with anger, with fleeing, with fighting, with depression, with apathy, with joy, etc... Our behavior and emotions are triggered to a large extent by our thoughts about the different aspects of our balance. In principle, we can influence these thoughts very well.

"Stress is in the mind of the beholder": **stress is what you think about it**. You can tip the balance completely by looking at the pandemic with very negative feelings, and negative magnifying glasses, by for instance continuously following the news items. That is of no use at all. The media need our attention and they like to get it with sensational news caused by gripping, mostly negative but extremely rare things. They do so because we are so sensitive to them; good news does not attract our attention enough.

Unfortunately, there is a fast-forward in our reflex-brain-system that makes us believe that things we can remember well, happen to us a lot. As a result, we intuitively think that what the media present to us happens more than what they don't write or talk about and that we for example think that more people are killed by sharks than by cows. As a result, when a few murders receive media attention, our gut feeling dictates us that the number of murders has increased, even if they decreased significantly.

"A cat has died of the coronavirus, even worse a sixteen-year-old died of it, or even worse a baby died of it." As a result, some people no longer dare to go outside with a baby or a teenager, while kids are more likely to die from an unfortunate fall in the bathroom than from the coronavirus. The media also like to enlarge the mistakes of our governments and look for culprits. However, in such a complex crisis, with so many unknown factors, your government has no choice but making choices between impossible dilemmas and making mistakes, hopefully while learning from the mistakes instead of looking for culprits. It is very much trial, error and learn for everybody.

The issue is simple: Good news does not sell because we are spontaneously attracted by bad news. As a result, even the best of our fact-checking media serve us a an overdoses of bad news. However, the anti-social media such as Facebook in particular, thrive on bad news because it makes us click, and that's how they make their money. They continuously and purposefully grab the attention of our primitive reflex-brain with messages, even unfiltered completely fabricated ones, that evoke negative emotions such as fear, anger and rage.

In the case of Covid-19, it's not so difficult to abuse our feelings of anxiety. Moreover, we are naturally more afraid of the unknown than of what we know and we try to understand things that sometimes the best scientists cannot explain. If anxious people can't understand what is happening they easily look for an easy culprit or resort to conspiracy theories because it gives the feeling that they understand what's happening. (You can read more about those primitive shortcuts in my book "BrainChains")

The solution: choose the way you look at things.

For your own mental health in this pandemic: stay away as much as possible from the antisocial media like Facebook. If you really can't live without, use them only to keep in touch with your inner circle of REAL friends and family. Never ever use them as a reliable source of news, for your own sake: please don't.

Even if you do not believe the dangerous avalanche of misinformation, you should limit your use of the antisocial media because of the continuous small self-injections of stress-inducing negative thoughts. Partly because of the way the media present the news, you think "What a blunder from the government that they didn't have those facial masks earlier", while you can also look at the same fact a different way like "How clever that the foreign affairs office could get a hold of 2.5 million facial masks that were ordered and held illegally by other countries". Is this naive? No, it is just a rational choice for the most healthy view.

Therefore, even if you mainly follow fact-checking media for your news, an urgent and important advice is to stay sane and reduce your stress is: don't listen/look/read the news more than twice a day.

Don't take part in that irrational, counterproductive and sometimes mean game of always looking for culprits. Looking for a single culprit you don't try to understand, you miss out on opportunities to learn. In such a unique, complex situation as this pandemic it is always a matter of "trial, error, debrief and adapt", for yourself, your family, your work, your government. Looking for a culprit in this unavoidable process of "trial and error", we miss out on the most important part: "debrief and adapt". It's a missed opportunity to learn and to become active and proactive and to instill progress and hope.

It is also important for your stress balance in this crisis that going along with that negative view of the matter has an additional negative weight on your own stress balance and that it may even prevent you from doing what you can or should do yourself.

Looking for a culprit is also an excuse for not doing what we can do in our own niche of control to stop the propagation of the virus. After the lockdown was introduced in Belgium, 50% of Belgians felt that the government should have acted sooner and stricter, but 85% kept shaking hands with friends and colleagues.

Know the facts and choose a reliable news source for your information, for example, https://coronavirus.jhu.edu/covid-19-basics/faq and https://coronavirus.jhu.edu/covid-19-basics/understanding-covid-19 . Put the COVID disaster, no matter how bad it is, in its rational context.

Why A Conspiracy Theorist Cannot Be Converted

The belief in conspiracy theories is centuries old and universal. They have always been there. The conspiring enemy is changing: Muslims, non-Muslims, Christians, heretics, Jews, pedophiles ... We've all had them before. In the past, however, these conspiracy theories were more regional straw fires, while they are now worldwide forest fires fanned and spread by the anti-social media. These conspiracy theories used to burn out because people were left exposed to other corrective information, but today the anti-social media encourages victims to dig deeper into their trap by only giving them information that confirms their belief.

The fact that these conspiracy theories are timeless indicates that they meet fairly basic needs, especially in uncertain times.

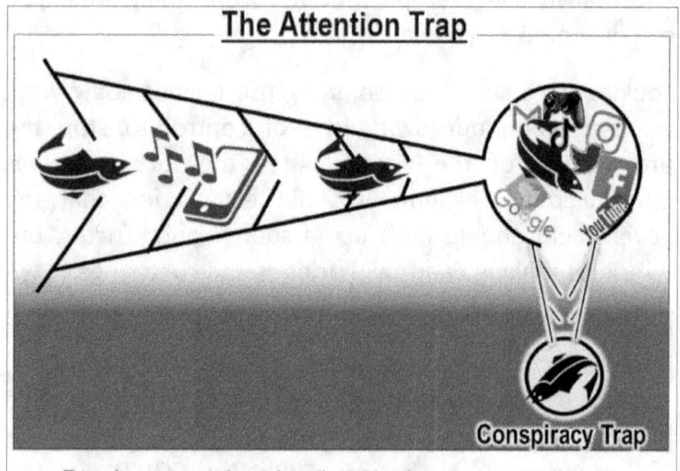

To make money antisocial media ruthlessly trap your attention with whatever it takes, even giant lies, especially by provoking anger and anxiety

The big advantage of believing in a conspiracy theory is that it offers guidance in a insane world. Thanks to the conspiracy theory, you understand what is happening, you have a simple all-encompassing explanation for a complex event that is difficult for even the smartest scientists to comprehend. Your unshakable belief gives you a sense of security and perspective. There is no risk that other information will make you doubt, because the anti-social media algorithms only give you information about what you already believe, reinforcing your belief with every click. Moreover, the algorithms are structured in such a way that once you have shown interest in a conspiracy theory, the algorithms automatically provide you with other conspiracy theories, so that it becomes increasingly clear to you that it is all a big conspiracy. That is your world view and that provides guidance.

A "good" conspiracy theory not only makes this complex incomprehensible world simple and understandable again. It also gives you a purpose, a perspective and a task, which is to convince others of the plot. You also feel superior to all those people who are so naive not to believe in the plot and that's a good feeling.

Moreover, the conspiracy theory also gives you the important feeling of belonging to a group of initiates that cling together well, partly because a conspiracy theory always creates a common enemy. Thanks to the anti-social media you now even have a worldwide network of people who think about it like you.

Belief in a conspiracy theory therefore has benefits for your stress balance. A major drawback, however, is that your belief in the plot makes you part of a huge network of virtual friends, but it threatens to alienate you from the real people around you. Another big drawback for your own stress balance is that those conspiracy theories cause nothing but negative emotions, because the anti-social media algorithms found that if their information scares you or angers you, you click a lot more and they earn more money with every click. The result: The more you look for information on the anti-social media, the more you only get information that reinforces your negative feelings.

Chronic negative feelings such as fear and anger cause a lot of negative stress and that is not good for your health.

Another disadvantage for yourself is that if you only get information through the anti-social media, you will no longer receive information that can adjust your opinion at least a little. Your opinion will become more and more oversimplified and rigid, and it will become impossible to escape over time. You have actually lost your freedom of thought.

There are, of course, also disadvantages for others and in particular for the enemy of a conspiracy theory.

So do not try to convince family members, friends or colleagues with rational arguments that they are wrong. Giving up the conspiracy theory causes too much uncertainty. Don't forget that you can't compete with the algorithms of anti-social media such as Facebook and YouTube. Even today, knowing full well what disasters they caused, they are unwilling to change their business model that spreads the anger and fear provoking misinformation worldwide, and that stimulates people to dig deeper into a trap of misinformation and blatant lies.

In the Corona crisis, the billion dollar earning algorithms of these anti-social media have literally become deadly. Not only because they spread fake news about the causes and treatment of the disease, but also because they opened the floodgates to the baseless, ignorant and life-threatening misinformation about vaccination. The anti-social media let this most dangerous fake news go viral, while originally it started with a small group of unhappy, ill-informed people. As a result, thousands of children are already dying unnecessarily from measles, a disease that was almost eradicated thanks to vaccination. But it's worse than that, because this baseless fear jeopardizes mass vaccination, the only solution we have to beat the coronavirus

So if a family member, friend, or co-worker has fallen into the trap of a conspiracy theory, you have no choice but to try to avoid the discussion about the plot and keep the relationship as good as possible, so that these people don't become completely isolated from their real life. social system. Don't feel superior, because it is clear that anyone, including the most clever of people, can accidentally fall into such a trap.

Stacking Stress

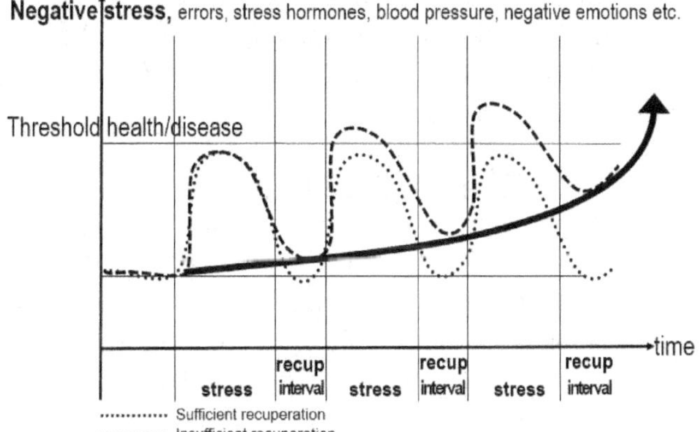

Healthy Stress Is Interval Stress

Healthy stress is interval stress. If we take regular recovery breaks we can cope with quite a lot of stress. The alternation between considerable stress and sufficient recovery makes us even stronger. The stress that makes us sick is chronic stress.

The solution: Divide your tasks as much as possible into continuous blocks per day and per week, with regular breaks (More about this in my book "BrainChains"). For yourself, but especially if you live with children: ensure regularity. A fixed, predictable daily schedule that fits in as much as possible with your life when not in lockdown. This predictability is important for everyone, but even more so for children.

Don't sit on each other's lips all the time, make sure there are fixed opportunities to take a break, to withdraw, and to rest mentally. Make sure you exercise sufficiently so that you are also physically tired, so you can sleep well and sufficiently. You don't need expensive equipment or fitness clubs to keep yourself moving every day. You can also start your fitness club with your family using creatively designed tools.

Focus On Your Niche Of Control

As for the **feeling of influencing that situation**, Epictetus (AD 55-135) sums it up nicely: "Suffering is the result of trying to influence that which we have no influence over and not doing what falls within our influence...and we are free to choose". Or as I once heard the Dalai Lama say, "In difficult situations. Think very carefully! If there's a solution, there's no reason to worry. If there really is no solution, then there's no reason to worry."

In other words: There's no point in worrying about things you can't control.

The solution: concentrate on things you do have an influence on and make an action plan.

Your 3 spheres of influence

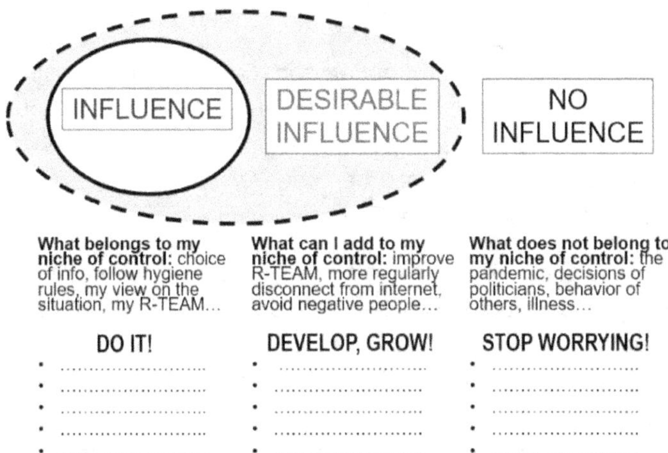

The more things you tackle, small and big, in your family role, your circle of friends, your neighborhood, the more you build on that vital feeling of having an impact on your situation; even if it all seems small compared to the disaster that Covid-19 causes. Don't underestimate what a positive influence it can have on yourself to cook something special, to do a long-delayed repair, finally read "BrainChains";-) or another book, to immerse yourself and your son in his beloved game that you never played with him, to yoga at home. On my bike ride, I just saw a young father jogging with his five-year-old daughter. She imitated him in earnest while he was stretching. They both enjoyed it.

Later I describe how important it is to divide your work into batches in order to be efficient. But dividing your time into batches and then more or less sticking to it also gives you a better sense of control over your day. Those more or less fixed routines give you a healthy steady rhythm, grip and predictability when all normal daily routines have disappeared.

Keep in mind that **following the Corona hygiene rules correctly also gives you a feeling of influence.** Your contribution seems minimal, but if everyone does it, those annoying rules can become less strict for everyone and it saves many human lives.

Choose a maximum of five action points and at the end of the day don't ask yourself the question "Did I do this today" five times, because there are always reasons why it didn't work out as planned. Rather ask yourself the question "Did I do my best to...". You take the responsibility to do your best, there is never an excuse for it, you always have an influence on that.

A special note for managers: too often an exaggerated need for being in control, totally ruins working from home for their employees. In the third chapter about working from home and zoom-stress I explain how co-workers can manage such a manager. Here I just want to emphasize that you can trust 90%, or even more, of the people when they work from home. Therefore it does not make sense and it is totally counterproductive to try control and micromanage the potential 10% who might abuse the situation, by creating a lot of unnecessary stress for the 90% and undermining the quality and quantity of their work. To succeed as a manager with a workforce working from home, you need two things: trust and transparency. And by the way, that's something you always need to be successful as a manager.

Develop Your Resources Proactively

What are my resources, which ones could you develop or promote? The most important are Resilience, Time, Expertise, Attention, and Material Resources.

The greater the resilience of a bow, the harder you can tension the bow: take good care of yourself.

Our resilience is determined by personal characteristics, by the degree to which our priorities are clear, by adequate assertiveness, by the way we deal with emotions, by our fitness (things like regular exercise or fitness, eating the right things, not smoking, alcohol consumption in moderation, etc.) All these aspects are extensively discussed in the book "Stress: Friend and Foe".

One factor that has an extraordinarily positive influence on your resilience is **having a good social support network** in which you can find both practical support for practical problems and emotional support. Let's not forget that human beings are herd animals. In fact, the human being is the most social animal on earth with a deep need to belong to the "tribe", to experience social contact in person. For so many people work is a very important source of social contact. For some who lack social contact in their private life, it is the most important source.

So this is a big challenge and sometimes a serious problem in times of lockdown. If you have neglected that network for a long time, for example by being too busy with your work or family, then all is not lost. Providing social support to others is also good for your own resilience.

If you want to support someone or strengthen the relationship: call. A telephone conversation has a much greater positive influence on the stress balance of the other person (and yourself) than just an email or text message. You can of course also offer real help and support and participate in initiatives of solidarity in your community.

You may keep or re-establish contact via the anti-social media, but stay in charge of those media. Use them only for social contact with people who are also important to you in your real life. Invest your time in people who really mean something to you or to whom you can really mean something. Above all, choose contact with positive friends. Chronically negative nags should be avoided, they don't do your stress balance any good. However, someone who wasn't negative in the past but is negative now, may be depressed. If it's someone you know quite well, keep in touch, and offer support.

Don't lose valuable social time with completely irrelevant information about completely irrelevant virtual "friends". Also, don't get caught up in the antisocial media's sneaky tricks to keep your attention, which will keep you from getting to the things and people that are really important and really good for you and the people in your real network. Set time limits for your social media usage.

High stress exposes your weaknesses. If it becomes too much for you, if you notice signs of stress in yourself or your housemates, if relationships become under too much tension, ask for help quickly, if necessary **ask for professional help**. Don't postpone it. There are plenty of services and counselors available by phone or video.

2. <u>How To Protect Your Think-Brain And Your Archiving Brain Against Your Reflex-Brain</u>

<u>Your Three Brains In A Nutshell</u>

There are three brain-networks (to simplify I call them often "brains") that play a role in thinking and making decisions. I describe these, and much more, in my comprehensive book "BrainChains" and its concise version "How To Unchain Your Brain"

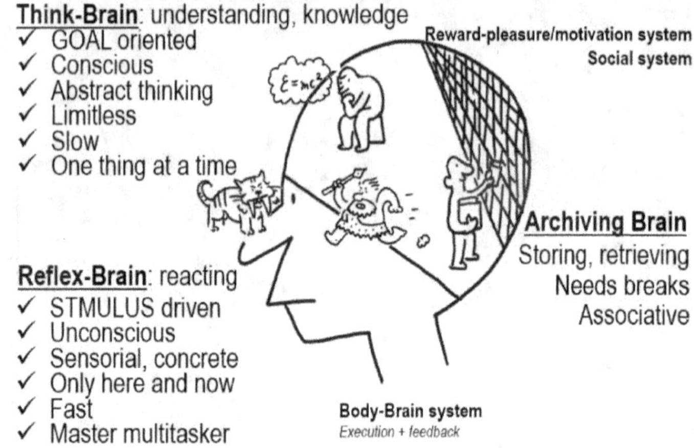

The first is the think-brain-network that developed very recently in evolution. That kind of brain is unique to humans. No other animal has the ability to think about things that are not present. To please animal lovers, let's say that dolphins, elephants, monkeys, pigeons, can do this a tiny little bit if you really stretch the definition, but we are the only animals who can really do abstract thinking. We humans can think back to the past and combine several memories from the past to find a solution for today or tomorrow. We can make plans for the future. We can think in terms, "what if?", we can postpone a decision, give it some more thought.

It's extraordinary what your thinking brain can do, but you can only properly focus on one thing at a time. Therefore, multitasking, doing two cognitive tasks at the same time is impossible. It is an illusion. This juggling of information takes time and energy, time you cannot spend on the tasks. If you try anyway, it costs you dearly in time, accuracy, memory, creativity, productivity, efficiency and stress. Don't forget that every interruption, every email, every tweet, every phone call you hear, is a switch. Every pop-up screen announcing an email causes a drop in concentration of two minutes, even if you ignore it. Compared to do one task at a time or doing one big chunk of a task at a time, multitasking takes more than double the time, causes errors and creates more stress.

The second network the reflex-brain-network, is evolutionary terms almost as old as animal existence. Very primitive animals that have grown a few hundred brain cells already develop reflexes. The world of the reflex-brain is here and now, all I experience now with all my senses. Our reflexbrain does not have to pay attention, its attention is effortlessly drawn by anything that's new, that's interesting (even if totally irrelevant), that provokes anxiety or anger, that's a signal of a group we want to belong to etc. etc. All the brain-mechanisms that the antisocial media like Facebook deliberately exploit to catch our attention permanently, to turn us into addicts and to make us click and work for them 2-3 hours a day for free, so that they can turn our attention into billions of revenue.

The third brain is the archiving brain that stores the information. Do you remember your teacher of first or second year of primary school? Did you ever need that information? And yet it is stored. Every single day you store billions bytes of information. This brain works in close cooperation with your think-brain. It's often called the default brain, because it works the hardest when your thinkbrain works less, takes a break or sleeps.

The Root Problem Is Always Being Connected

The opportunity to be always connected is fantastic for our brainwork. However, always being connected is a disaster for your brainwork. In my book "Brainchains" and it's compact version "How to unchain your brain" I explain in depth the reasons why you can never realize the best of your brain if you are always connected. There are many reasons for this.

The three most important ones are

First of all that being always connected seduces you to multitask all the time and that is a total disaster for your intellectual productivity, accuracy, creativity, memory and stress.

Secondly that always begin connected creates chronic stress, because you are always on alert and because it makes you so f&^%*#@ inefficient that you need much more time to do a worse job.

Thirdly that you tend to stay involved with screens way to late, get insufficient sleep, which is very bad for your intellectual productivity, accuracy, creativity, memory, stress and health.

The Only Solution: Batch-Tasking

The solution is batch-tasking or batch-processing.

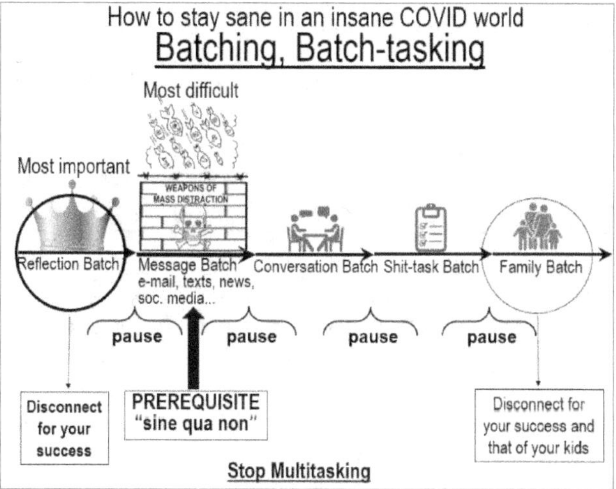

The first and most important batch is an ironclad do-not-disturb cage around your important brainwork. Continuously checking your e-mail and social media is the worst enemy of your thinking brain. The other deadly enemy is an open plan office layout, but for many of you in covid-times the problem is rather to organize your work at home in a brain-friendly way.

The second and most difficult batch to achieve the first is that you need to build a shelter to protect yourself from the *weapons of mass distraction*. The never ending stream of interesting but mainly irrelevant information. To this end, you plan a block of time four times a day in which you do nothing but respond to all possible messages. Ideally, you have set up your messaging system so that most irrelevant information no longer reaches you.

Then you also need to create a batch for conversations and one for little shit-tasks that also might otherwise interrupt your thinkwork batch.

Don't forget to finish each batch with a break so that your archiving brain can store and organize the information and trigger creative insights.

The Most Important Batch: Your Thinkwork Batch

To be productive and creative, you have to protect your fantastic but vulnerable and easily tired thinking-brain against all the endless distractions that hijack your primitive, tough and tireless reflex-brain.

Therefore you plan regular slots of disconnected time for uninterrupted, focused work or conversations. Ruthlessly organize your working environment to eliminate distractions. First of all you have to disconnect from the endless stream of messages. If you have a door, close it. If you don't have a door, look for a space that has one or put a screen around your workspace, put earplugs in your ears and a big headphone on your head, it doesn't even have to work, but it functions as a strong "do not disturb" message. Put up a "do not disturb" sign, switch-off your phone and all the pop-up screens and beeps on your computer. Put a clever do-not disturb message on your voicemail and out of office email. Most important and most difficult: disconnect from all messages.

The minimum time you should be disconnected is twice a day for 45 minutes each. Fight for it tooth and nail. You will have to be creative, relentless and even ruthless about this, towards your environment and towards yourself.You may forget every single piece of advice in this book, but if you implement just this one, it will significantly improve your intellectual productivity.

Finish it off with a break for archiving the information you just processed. The more difficult the work you did, the longer the break should be.

The Most Difficult Batch: Putting All "Weapons Of Mass Distraction" In Message Batches

If you ever want to restore the full power of your thinking brain, you have to be in control of your ICT and especially your phone, instead of the other way around. You have to break that most important brainchain. This the most crucial action you can take to liberate your brainpower.

Period.

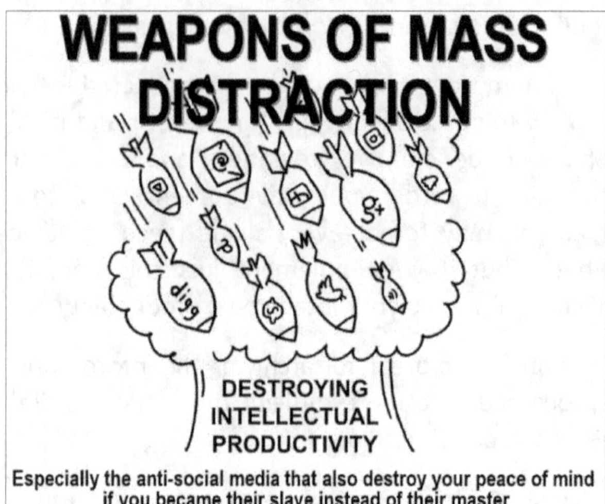

Especially the anti-social media that also destroy your peace of mind
if you became their slave instead of their master

You should handle your emails, messages, social media and news in as few batches per day as possible. For most people this is four batches per day. You must put an impenetrable wall around this batch: don't let them distract you outside these batches: lock them up. You should manage these batches with the attitude of a real professional, not as an addicted consumer. YOU ought to decide how much time you will spend on them, where you do it and when. You should do this batch in a professional environment with professional hardware and software, NOT on your smartphone with two clumsy thumbs on a Tom Thumb screen. Your phone is a gadget and an emergency tool. It's totally unfit for efficient professional work.

Eliminate all seductive sirens that lure you to your inbox, where the ship of your creativity will become stranded: eliminate all beeps and pop up screens. They should not decide when you look at messages, you should. Unsubscribe from all the automatic messages from the big time-wasters of email, social media and news. Learn how simple it is to make your e-mail program file CC-mails automatically. Don't use your inbox as a to-do list but put important work at once in your agenda and unimportant chores on a list for your shit-task-batch (see below).

You will be astonished how much less time you will spend on your emails and how much better they will be, if you do them in batches and then stop connecting the rest of the day. This is very difficult in the beginning, but once you get used to it, it makes a huge difference for your productivity, creativity and stress.

So many people who did accomplish noted their increased efficiency with a very surprised "I have so much more time now".

Don't Let Unplanned Chats And Shit-Tasks Ruin Your Important Brainwork

Shit-tasks are little tasks you don't like, and can't delegate. You are frustrated when you get them and you try to postpone them, but they keep nagging at you from the back of your mind. Way too often you have to set aside much more important work, because suddenly a postponed little shit-task became urgent.

The solution is to plan a shit-task-batch every week. Then, when you get a shit-task you can put it on a list and schedule a time slot once a week to handle them all. If you do that, you get less frustrated when you receive one and it won't keep nagging at you because you planned a time to handle it. Hence, there is less risk they will disturb important work. Moreover, doing one of these tasks does not give you much satisfaction, but when you clean up a heap of them, especially just before the weekend, it gives you a good feeling

Give Your Brain The Pauses And Sleep It Needs To Excel.

For your archiving-brain to archive, for your thinking brain to recuperate and to restore your stress-balance, you should have a break after every single task that requires thinking, attention and concentration. You should not skip lunch, or continue to work while having lunch. Having a proper lunch-break, where you disconnect from work, is an excellent investment in the quantity and quality of your brainwork. Taking a break behind your screen surfing on the antisocial media is a break, but for your brain (and the rest of your body) it's a very poor one. Get away from behind your desk, do something different, something physical like cleaning a room or better even, get out of the house and go for a brisk walk.

Working extra hours does not increase productivity or creativity; on the contrary, it decreases it. Stop the work-day in time to allow time to recuperate. Always being connected creates the risk that all boundaries between work and private life disappear, and working from home makes it almost unavoidable, but do your best to keep boundaries as much as possible. Reorganize your life around the results of the two sleep-tests . For your biological clock, you should start with getting up every day at the same time. If you need more sleep on the weekends, go to bed earlier. The feeling of needing more sleep in the weekend to recuperate from the week is a clear signal that you are sleep deprived: very bad for your

<u>WHAT IS ENOUGH SLEEP FOR YOU</u>

<u>Test 1</u>. The hours of sleep you need so that you don't need to sleep-in in the week-ends

<u>Test 2</u>. The hours of sleep you need to get through the workday feeling rested, lucid and alert <u>without stimulants</u>
(no caffeine, no coffee, no black or green tea, no coke, no energy (*LOL!*) drinks, no amphetamines, cocaine etc...)

-**Without symptoms of sleep-debt** such as:
 difficult getting out of bed, feeling sleepy, feeling tired, nodding off, feeling drowsy while driving!, needing a nap, craving for junk food or sugar after you had a normal meal, sleeping extra hours in weekend

-**Without brain symptoms** such as:
 Concentration↓ Memory ↓ Patience ↓ Feeling for nuance ↓ Insight ↓ Judgement ↓ Creativity ↓ Multitasking ↓ Decision capability ↓ Depression ↑ Moodiness ↑ Happiness ↓ Enthusiasm ↓ Sexual desire ↓

Warning: the first 14 days without caffeine you may have withdrawal symptoms, such as lack of concentration, headaches, feeling feverish, feeling tired.

thinkbrain. Ideally, you should plan all important, difficult or complex brainwork in the morning after a good night's sleep and before you look at your messages. That way you will get the maximum benefit from the important work your archiving brain did during the time you were asleep to prepare you for the day. You can find many more tips in "BrainChains".

3. <u>How to Avoid Zoom-stress</u>

Are you, like most people, much more exhausted after a day with many video-conferences than after a full day of in person interactions? How come and what can you do about it?

On my computer I installed Skype, Zoom, Starleaf, Webex, Teams, Facetime and Whatsapp to continue collaborating with my clients. The fact that video conferencing technology is now widely available to everyone and everywhere is really fantastic. Who could have thought this possible only ten years ago? Without that technology, the impact of the COVID pandemic on work and school would have been much worse. The pandemic forced a lot of reluctant people and companies to discover the important advantages of the videoconference tools and the possibilities of working from home. Yet, at the same time, we all discovered the limitations, disadvantages and stress of working from home. People spontaneously started talking about "zoom stress".

An important part of the zoom-stress is not caused by virtual work itself, but by having to work digitally without being really well prepared, with insufficient time to adapt, with children and an equally tense partner around you, in a continuous crisis state, along with the anxiety of experiencing a global pandemic, of a lockdown, of the fate of COVID patients amongst family and friends, of the fear of infection or contamination of loved ones , or of losing our job. This undermines some very basic human needs of social contact and intimate relationships, status, a sense of mastery, of control, financial security. As a result, many people carry a heavier burden than usual and sometimes that digital hassle, and the lack of the social support of their colleagues or manager, is just too much.

Knowing a little more about the impact of this way of working will help you to cope with it in a more productive and healthy way. There are social and technical issues to take into consideration. The social issues can be dealt with your stress-balance in mind. I'd like to explain some of the technical issues and solutions.

Tricks The Technology Plays On Stress And Feeling Of Wellbeing

It took hundreds of thousands of years for the human race to develop the flabbergasting brain we have today. Above I described three brain networks that help us to think, decide and act. But to understand how we deal with virtual contact you need to understand that we also have developed a social-brain-network making us the most social animal in the world. Now we can even have social visual contact with people on the other side of the world.

In the course of time the human race developed a wide range of innate, lifesaving, social reflexes to unconsciously process very subtle nonverbal clues very fast. These allow us to instantly differentiate between people like me and people not like me, people I can trust or not, people that are safe or dangerous. The problem is that these signals, and especially the most important facial cues, are sometimes distorted by the technology. We only see a face instead of a whole body and we see it flat instead of in three dimensions. As a result our impression of the other person is unconsciously biased, usually in a negative way, not only making spontaneous distrust more likely, but also creating more stress. For example, not receiving any non-verbal feedback during an interaction is very stressful especially if the interaction is important. Many researchers demonstrated this for example by measuring the stress of babies, children and adults during an interaction when the other person freezes all her nonverbal facial reactions.

This is part of the explanation why we are often less stressed in an audio tele-conference than in front of a wall of motionless faces staring at us. Even if we feel not consciously threatened, unconsciously our reflex social-brain triggers typical physiological stress reactions. You certainly have experienced this when a motionless "poker face" or a group of poker faces is used to create a feeling of anxiety in horror or crime movies. We intuitively know our hero is in an a dangerous situation when the other persons' faces stay immobile. Our conscious rational brain knows it is only a movie, but our unconscious reflex brain, reacts with all the signals of thrill and fear.

Moreover, the close-up video puts people's faces so big so close, that it feels like invading your privacy-bubble and might feel threatening for your reflex-brain, even if your think-brain rationally knows it's only a video.

Another important   cue that's missing in video-conferencing is eye-contact. In normal life we are suspicious of a person avoiding eye contact. Of course we all rationally know that the lack of eye contact in a videoconference is a mere technological issue, but our irrational reflexbrain might still instill a little bit of that primitive innate suspicion, just enough to make the conversation a little less trusting. On the other hand, when people do their best to give an impression of eye-contact, by looking all the time straight into the camera, this does not feel safe either for cave(wo)man inside each of us.

A more subtle issue, that has a negative impact on the non-verbal feedback, is when there is a desynchronization of the sound and the video. Even when the discrepancy is minimal our reflex brain will have difficulty connecting the words and the nonverbal cues, causing more stress and increasing a tendency to distrust the information. Even if the delay is less than a second our reflex-brain will tend to see the other as less trustworthy, less interested and less friendly.

No wonder that video-negotiations run a higher risk of failing, given these innate trust undermining tendencies caused by the technology, that make it much more difficult to correctly assess each other's emotions.

And of course there is also the nuisance when we have to fiddle around with the technology to show something, compared to a real meeting were we just show the object or turn our screen to the others or simply push the button of our ClickShare.

Be that as it may, there are quite a few things you can do, regardless of that context, to improve your stress-balance while working and meeting from home.

<u>Solutions Within Your Own Sphere Of Influence</u>

<u>Keep boundaries around your different life spheres</u>

In "BrainChains" I explain why it is so important to guard the boundaries between the different domains of your life. The five boundaries are work/private, public/private, real/virtual, present/absent, body/mind. These boundaries do not function like impenetrable concrete walls, they are always somewhat flexible. However, when you work from home the first three often tend to weaken or disappear. It is not only better for your batch-tasking to keep these domains as separated as possible. It is also better for your stress-balance and your mental health, not the least because organizing then gives you a feeling of control.

<u>Your Working Environment</u>

Since COVID is here to stay for a while and since working from home will become common, invest in creating a professional context for working from home: a large screen, a comfortable keyboard and headphones and a good ergonomic office chair. For 30 € you can even buy a little adaptor/docking station, so that you can easily plug your laptop in and out of your home setup. If you really can't afford a big screen, buy a separate keyboard and mouse. It allows you to put the screen of your laptop on eyelevel. This 20, - € is a very small investment to avoid stress in your back and neck and to improve your video-conferences.

Invest also in the best broadband connection you can get. You probably have already one for streaming entertainment. If not get one. Many employers are willing to pay their part of it.

Try to organize a neutral background for your video conferences, so that when you are speaking, the attention of the listener (s) goes to you and not to your living room or bookshelf. Avoid backlight, because when your face is n the shadow the reflexbrain of the others will signal "don't trust".

Many people have virtual meetings with a laptop where the camera is above or below the screen. If the camera is too close, you only see their head and it gives the impression that they look at your belly or your crown. You get kind of used to it but it is not ideal and believe it or not: it has a negative influence on the quality of the conversation. If the best you have is a laptop, place your laptop screen at eye level on a box or a stack of books and place it as far away from you as comfortable for you to see your screen. If you look at your built-in camera from further away, the eye contact is a bit more natural. When people can see each other's upper body and arms and not just a talking head, this improves the conversation. Therefore, a separate camera, with a zoom-lens and a better mike are excellent investments. With these you can move the camera further away and zoom in or out. I put a separate camera on a tripod, in front of my big screen about the distance I need to look like a TV presenter.

If possible, create a working corner that is separated from the living room. If it's a corner of your bedroom, it's easier to get the message out to family members that you shouldn't be disturbed.

An apparent detail that sometimes has more of an influence than you think: if you work from home, dress just like you would in the office. You just feel different, more professional, in work clothes than in a jogging suit, quickly covered by a shirt or blouse. Maybe you are an exception, but try experimenting with it anyway. Moreover, it signals to other people in the house that you are at work.

Make sure you have enough breaks between meetings and move around during those breaks. If you can't go outside just do sit-ups, push-ups, step-ups, just run up and down the stairs or use your fitness machine a few minutes, if you have one.

Your interaction with your camera and the video screen.

First of all, stop looking at yourself. Once you made certain the camera settings and background are OK , hide your own video. In a real conversation you don't look at yourself in a mirror all the time! You shouldn't look at yourself in a video meeting either. It is an unnecessary, energy wasting and stress increasing distraction and nobody knows what impact it has on you and your self-consciousness when you are looking in that video-mirror several hours a day. Moreover, when you look at yourself you run a greater risk of having an irrational negative impression of your interventions.

Besides it is embarrassing to see how often people start grooming behavior as if they are looking in a mirror, forgetting that a whole bunch of people are looking from behind that "mirror" while you are primping.

In some videoconference apps it is possible to enable a hide self feature. If yours has one, use it. If not you might use a little app I use "deskpin" that allows one to keep a window on top. This way I can make a little notepad window, and put that on top of anything else, and I can easily swipe it to the side, like al little curtain, to check if everything is OK.

Secondly, don't stare at the camera all the time. In an in-person conversation you don't stare at the person all the time. No, you switch all the time between a brief eye-contact and looking in other directions. Do the same when having a video conversation.
When you are giving a more formal presentation it is OK to look more straight ahead into the camera, as a TV-presenter does.

Next, move your camera away from you, so that on your camera the distance looks like the one you would have around a meeting table. When people can see your hands, your non-verbal communication becomes richer and they can see you are taking notes when you are not looking at them via de camera, which resolves the eye contact dilemma (see below).
Importantly, you stay out of the "psychological interpersonal distance bubble" people need to feel comfortable. In a real conversation, you are not always in close up staring at each other. Unless you are lovers, this close distance is threatening and may still be on a subliminal level.
Imagine you enter an small elevator at work with five people you vaguely know and they all keep staring at you from such a close distance, and they keep staring at you,

even when somebody else in the elevator speaks. How would you feel? Certainly not very comfortable. Well, that's another reason why videoconferences are so tiring. Rationally, your thinkbrain knows of course that the situation in a videoconference is different and is not threatening, but unconsciously your primitive reflexbrain is continuously pressing your alarm buttons.

If you put your camera farther away, eye-contact looks more natural, especially if you are not continuously staring at the camera, but once in while look away from the camera, as you would do in an in-person conversation. But that creates a bit of a dilemma, because in a real meeting people would know that you are looking out of the window, at another person or at your notes. In a zoom meeting they have no clue. When you look at the left that looks like it is in the direction of the (video of) the person at the left of your video, but it might also give the impression that you are looking at another person in your room, invisible for the people in the virtual meeting. My solution is to take a thinking/listening posture looking slightly down, chin on hand, while regularly looking briefly upward straight into the camera, or to take notes (or do as if) and to regularly look up into the camera.

If you are farther away from the camera and you want to emphasize something you can always briefly get closer to the camera with your face (don't forget that inbuilt cameras are rather wide angle and distort your face when you get close).

During meetings, take notes with pen and paper to keep you focused. This interrupts the staring and being stared at, in an acceptable way, especially if people can see that you are taking notes.. Moreover, you remember and integrate information better than when you take notes with your tablet or laptop. By the way, in in–person meetings or courses, taking notes with paper and pen is also more efficient than doing this on a laptop. If your camera shows more than only your head, people will see that you are taking notes and that you are not just losing interest and doing something else.

Since the nonverbal cues are often shrunk to the level of being invisible, don't count on your usual subtle nonverbal feedback. You'll have to exaggerate them somewhat. If you agree and want to support the speaker: nod visibly, if you disagree: shake "no" visibly, if you want to say something, raise your hand.

Recurrently hide the conference window from your view for two reasons.
First because of the very tiring trouble our brain has with the increased "cognitive load" of all the subtle "wrong" or meaningless non-verbal messages you get from a screen full of videos.
Second because all those close-up faces, continuously staring at you, create unnecessary stress.
Therefore you should regularly take a mini-video-break from the visual non-verbal chaos on your screen by minimizing the whole video window, to follow the meeting with audio only while looking at a peaceful landscape on your desktop or in a photoapp.

Take micro-breaks

If you turn off your own camera, while listening, you can stand up, look out of your window, do a few stretching exercises, breathing exercises or even a few push-ups, sit-ups or other physical exercises.

These micro-breaks to move around are not only important for you thinking brain and especially its creativity, but also for the rest of your body. When we are in a videoconference, trying to stay at our best within the camera range, we become basically frozen, for hours in a row sometimes. The lack of physical movement in a regular meeting is already often challenging for our body, but in a video conference it becomes a real problem, especially if you spend many hours a day behind your screen in front of a camera. Hence, try to loosen up in video-conferences and change your body position often. You will see that this comes more natural when the camera is farther away from you. Then, have microbreaks and use the time between meetings to do some physical exercise. I got fond of the 7 minute workouts the easier one at https://nyti.ms/3i4XQga and the more difficult one at http://nyti.ms/3I6wKqw

Don't multitask

Teleconferencing makes it extremely tempting to do other things during a meeting, under the illusion that we can do two things at the same time. This not only increases the stress, it also greatly undermines the quality of meetings. In "BrainChains" and "How to unchain your brain", I explain in detail how horribly inefficient this kind multitasking is. Moreover, if you are busy with emails during a meeting, you miss a lot of information, you remember much less, you even hear things that have not been said and it is much more tiring for your brain and your creativity. Hence, during a meeting, life or virtual, your smartphone should be off. If the meeting is really boring it is better for your brain to daydream and much better to discuss with your manager and colleagues how to avoid these meetings or parts of meetings.

If the video quality becomes bad, delayed or shaky turn it off immediately and go on with audio. Better no visible face than a bad one or an immobile one (except when it is clearly a photo to show you are still connected) Moreover without video the audio often improves and you will be more comfortable, less stressed.

Disable video as much as possible

Last but not the least, even with the best of efforts, videoconferencing will always be more stressful, and the issue is exactly the "effort". First of all we have to continuously pretend we are paying full attention; a degree and a duration of attention that is unsustainable. Moreover, in in-person conversations all the very efficient non-verbal communication comes natural, without effort. Some of our reading of that behavior and our reactions are innate, others are so well learned habits that they become automatic. However, to get the best out of a videoconference we have to do an effort to do a lot of things that do not come natural, like looking straight into a camera once in a while as if you were looking at a person, exaggerating non-verbal feedback a little, speak a little louder that in a live conversation, not worrying about all those people staring in your face, etc... Luckily enough, when you do this a lot, it becomes a new habit, it becomes more automatic and "natural", and will cost less and less energy. However, don't underestimate the impact of video-conferencing on the spontaneous innate tendencies of our reflexbrain.

It is obvious that it is not the "electronic" conferencing that is the problem, but the video. Hence you may think: " Then, why would we go through all that trouble if we can have just phone conferences" and that is indeed the right question and the right answer. Because something is technically possible does not mean it is necessarily better. That is true about so many things, like taking notes on a laptop instead of with pen and paper. Indeed, for most meetings video has more disadvantages (eg. exhaustion!) than advantages.

> **The best way to avoid video-stress is to stop the video when it does not add value**

It is most often not necessary at all to always add the additional stress of having a video-conference, when a phone-conferences is much more efficient and less stressful. I hate to sound like a luddite because I love the technology and it certainly saved many of us in these corona times, but it is evident that the best way to avoid zoom-stress is to stop zooming all the time and use phone-conferences, unless you have solid reasons to think that a phone conference can't do the job.

You could also opt for a hybrid conference, especially in these pandemic times, where you open the meeting in video-mode briefly to greet and check-in and have some small-talk, then disable the camera's, and only use them (the whiteboard or the sharing mode) when you want to show something. You may then want to use the video-mode again to say goodbye.

Solutions For Which You Need Others

Make crystal-clear agreements with your housemates, so that you have disruption-free working time. This is not always easy, especially when the children are also at home. If you sit in front of your computer with your headphones, it must be a signal to everyone that you should not be disturbed. Be creative. Like Jenny, a single mother who agreed to take turns with her neighbor looking after their children, so that they each were better able to work from home undisturbed. If there really is no other solution, let your children play more with a tablet or phone than normally. Everybody who read my book "BrainChains" knows that I fight against letting kids too much connected to screens, but necessity breaks the law.

Keep video meetings as short as few and short as possible. They are too tiring.

Refuse meetings outside office hours unless there is no other option due to time differences. Discuss this with your colleagues and managers.

With people you already know, you can also opt for regular phone-conferences as they are less tiring. You are used to that, you know the limits and the possibilities, you know what to expect. Sometimes I start with video to greet each other, check in and then continue with audio only. If necessary, we can then return to video with one click to show something on the screen.

Experiment with this.. Be flexible. It's not because technology makes videoconferencing possible, that it is always the best solution.

Also for many managers, having their employees working from home was new. The good ones quickly discovered that you can trust people, that most people work as well and many even more or more efficient from home. The engagement surveys often show an increase in engagement. They also discovered that zoom-meetings demand more facilitating from the manager, among other things because introverts and women run the risk of being ignored, overruled or interrupted even more than in live meetings. They follow the adage "be in command not in control". They also care for the circumstances in which their employees work and invest in good broadband connections, big monitors, docking stations, headphones and other practical needs.

Managers with too much ego become insecure at the thought that they can be missed. Managers who like to keep everything under control or the so inefficient and demotivating micromanagers, become very insecure and even anxious with all their collaborators out of sight, working from home (although of course they will never admit it). As a result, in uncertain times they are inclined to pull the reins even harder and to maintain control by organizing many unnecessary, too large and too long video meetings.

Protest and negative feedback make these insecure managers even more insecure, making them want to control everything even more. Try to guide them (together with a few like-minded team members) in a positive, supportive way in small steps. More with the idea "How can we steer him in small steps, in a way in which he feels supported and learns to trust us and to let go".

In a team the team-members solved this by convincing their stressed controlling manager that they missed his substantive input, because he was too distracted by the process and the technical aspects of electronic meetings. They offered that someone on the team would take care of the technology and someone else would the process and the agenda. The latter, in effect, took the reins with a stricter and timed agenda, making meetings much shorter and preparing parts in smaller groups. In order to give the manager the feeling of control he so desperately sought, everyone told at the start of the small and large meetings, in two sentences, what she had been doing since the last meeting. The manager relaxed, gradually lost the need to attend every sub-meeting and became as inspiring as he was before he was promoted to be manager.

Of course most managers and employees miss live contact and for a lot of work and meetings it still is the most efficient way of collaborating. All surveys show, however, that for the future most employees would prefer the best of two worlds , and work in a hybrid work situation, combining working from home and in the office. We all learned the hard way that this is indeed a perfect solution for a lot of office work.

Conclusion: Push Your Pause Button

When you are aware of signals telling you the pandemic got you out of balance, take a short break to reflect on two figures your stress-balance and your resilience graph.

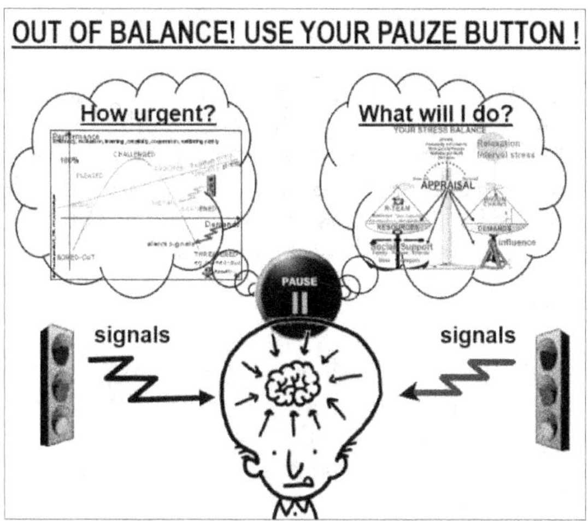

Then posit yourself on the resilience graph. This will tell you how urgent it is to take action. The deeper down on the right, the more urgent. Then have a look at your stress-balance and decide in what area you could or should intervene to restore your balance. If you do a lot of videoconferencing, do it as a professional.

You are lucky that scientist developed excellent vaccines so fast. That's your light at the end of the tunnel.

Good luck!

Theo

Readers' comments about "BrainChains"

Stunning work, aggregating the best and newest research
to create a User Manual for Your Brain! Whether all the
new tech is leveraged as a positive tool or allowed to
seduce us into numb- and dumbness is a fine line, and
Theo delineates that with brilliance. Read at your peril.
David Allen

Excellent book on productivity. If you have read David
Allen's Getting Things Done this book will be beneficial to
comprehend the whole system and why we do what we do.
Theo Compernolle's work is based on scientific research
and backs up his arguments in style. If there is one thing
you should take from BrainChains "Do not use your phone
while driving"
Addo General Mrch

I'm so glad I got my hands on this book. Forget all the
other business books, tips and theories which everybody
else uses, THIS is the book that will separate you away
from the herd and should be read before anything else.
This book will be kept on my desk instead of my
bookshelf, as a constant reminder.
NoName

In a few words: an amazing book. Loved reading it. The
author knows very well how to explain this matter in an
open end very comprehensible way. I look at my laptop in
a different way now. Must read!
4bozzza

This is one of those books that do have impact on your
habits … at least for me it did and that is I think the
biggest value a book can have…
Joanne

… an easy to read "page turner"… which I feel everyone
in the "connected" world should read.
Dave Scott, President

Top experience. Extended documentation.Accessible reading of "scientific" topics. Really professional. Appreciate the style and art of communication of the author. Congratulations. Excellent buy and investment.
Jean-Paul Antonus

"… a compelling, meticulously researched, and cleverly illustrated case against the twin tyrannies of hyperconnectivity and multitasking… also shows how to free ourselves from them"
Nélida and Jorge Colapinto

It is amazing (and disturbing) that what Theo writes of is so little known and/or poorly embraced by the business world. … Yet the working practices encouraged by firms, and societies as a whole serve to squander our IQ, EQ and SQ and foster burnout, unrealised potential and underperformance...
And the hyperconnectivity of recent years brought about by the smartphone has magnified the problem multiple-fold.
Congratulations to Theo for bringing this issue into the open with such a well-evidenced, thoughtful and readable analysis.
L. Watson

Excellent Book. I was addicted to "multitasking" and had trouble concentrating in longer tasks… Can honestly say that this book has changed me for the better!It is written in a very readable fashion and contains practical tips on how to make you brain work better and more efficiently. It's a kind of "User manual to your brain". How to use it correctly to gain the most stress free productivity…
Jose Rivero

Being filled all the time by all kinds of electronic information every day, I often feel myself lost in this "ICT world". How can we live and what shall we live as human? This book shows me a so powerful human brain ... Looking inside into my brain, I get my idea to have my life back under my own control, just like what is said in the

last poem: Recapture time to love and be loved, it is the keystone of happiness and resilience: yours and theirs.
Wei TAO, Business Information Manager

Wow. 6/12 into purchase of this book is still being pulled on and off my shelf. An amazing insight into our brain- possibly the best computer we will ever have the pleasure of owning! I've Learned lots already from this entertaining academic. Enlightening.
S.A.W. Bristol UK

Brilliant book and explodes all the rubbishy myths about multitasking
10HS

… blending his best knowledge in medical sciences and leadership development to give us a real eye opener on how our brain is working (or not) in our new environment.
Serge Zimmerlin. Group Vice President

The book was a revelation for me and helped me better understand why people do what they do in a health & safety context. An essential and easy read for practical people, who want to know how people work and what can be practically done to maximize their efficiency and reduce human error"
Malc Staves Global Health & Safety Director

… Innovations that work are selected and thrive, but some, like IT and hyperconnectedness, overshoot and threaten to become runaway phenomena. It took Prof. Compernolle's unique synthesis of brain science, expertise in human behavior and therapeutical skills to also provide remedies and to progress from Drucker's 'knowledge work' to Compernolle's 'brainwork'.
Prof. Jan Bernheim
A MUST READ for managers overall, but especially for responsible HR managers as the productivity of esp. white- collar employees is truly at risk in the 'Anytime, Anyplace' connected world of today. The research and in-practice evidence is overwhelming why we should not multitask,

always be connected or take short cuts on our sleep. I compare the impact of this book to the "Shallows: what the internet does to our brains" by N.Carr.
I have changed my personal habits immediately and now also inspire people around me at work and in my private life to do the same.
Philippe

It's obvious that our best tool to work and live it's our brain but unfortunately we often forget the way to use it correctly. Theo, in the funniest way I know, has found the right way to open my mind and improve my daily performance. Reading this book you will know how many mistakes make every day avoiding to use our brain correctly and how much time/money we could save hearing our body signals.
Ferdinand

"…Multitasking is impossible! Understanding and accepting this, helped me to refocus on tasks which matters and to rediscover my creativity. I used the short MULTITASKING test in my meetings in our global organization. It's exciting to see everywhere the "aha"-effect, the epiphany!"
Dr. Peter zum Hebel, Vice President

An absolute must if we want to safeguard or recover our brain's full capacity, productivity and creativity. A wise lesson to better master the ever growing number of addictive ICT-tools, thus improving our quality of life both at home and at work, and, who knows, even saving lives. And finally, a plea for more direct and true relationships in the real world instead of losing precious time in a mostly shallow virtual world
Prof Gino Baron

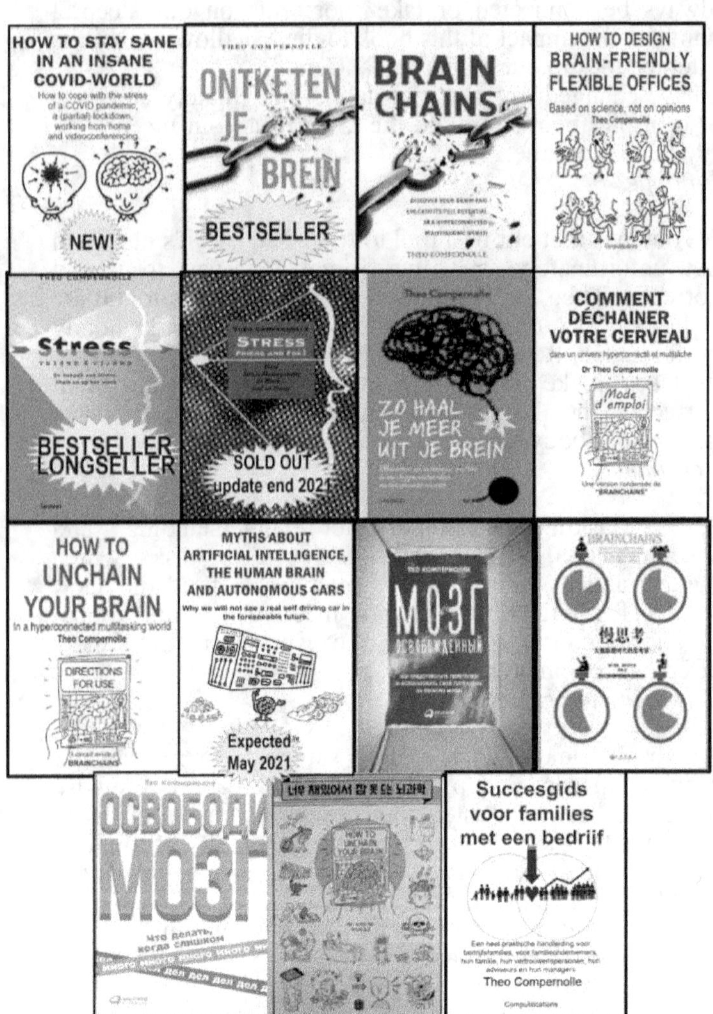

HOW TO STAY SANE IN AN INSANE COVID-WORLD
How to cope with the stress of a COVID pandemic, a (partial) lockdown, working from home and videoconferencing
NEW!
THEO COMPERNOLLE
ONTKETEN JE BREIN
BESTSELLER
BRAIN CHAINS
THEO COMPERNOLLE
HOW TO DESIGN BRAIN-FRIENDLY FLEXIBLE OFFICES
Based on science, not on opinions
Theo Compernolle
Stress
BESTSELLER LONGSELLER
STRESS
SOLD OUT
update end 2021
Theo Compernolle
ZO HAAL JE MEER UIT JE BREIN
COMMENT DÉCHAINER VOTRE CERVEAU
dans un univers hyperconnecté et multitâche
Dr Theo Compernolle
Mode d'emploi
"BRAINCHAINS"
HOW TO UNCHAIN YOUR BRAIN
In a hyperconnected multitasking world
Theo Compernolle
DIRECTIONS FOR USE
BRAINCHAINS
MYTHS ABOUT ARTIFICIAL INTELLIGENCE, THE HUMAN BRAIN AND AUTONOMOUS CARS
Why we will not see a real self driving car in the foreseeable future.
Expected May 2021
МОЗГ
BRAINCHAINS
慢思考
ОСВОБОДИ МОЗГ
Что делать, когда слишком
HOW TO UNCHAIN YOUR BRAIN
Succesgids voor families met een bedrijf
Theo Compernolle
Compublications